ESSENTIAL

Core

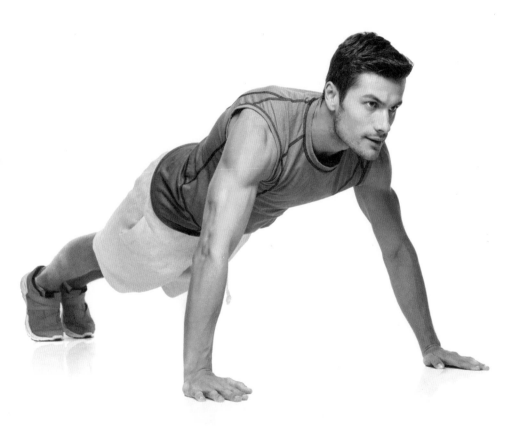

BluSky
PUBLISHERS.com

Published in North America by BluSky Publishers in association with Hinkler Books Pty Ltd 2016

First published by Hinkler Books Pty Ltd 2016
45–55 Fairchild Street
Heatherton Victoria 3202 Australia
www.hinkler.com.au

Text © Hinkler Books Pty Ltd 2012
Design © Hinkler Books Pty Ltd 2012, 2016

Created by Moseley Road Inc.
Editorial director: Lisa Purcell
Art director: Brian MacMullen
Cover and internals designer: Sam Grimmer
Photographer: Jonathan Conklin Photography, Inc.
Author: Hollis Lance Liebman
Models: Hollis Lance Liebman, Cori D. Cohen
Illustrator: Hector Aiza/3DLabz
Inset illustrations: Linda Bucklin/Shutterstock.com,
page 5 FXQuadro/Shutterstock.com,
page 6 Christopher Edwin Nuzzaco/Shutterstock.com,
page 7 Darrin Henry/Shutterstock.com
Prepress: Graphic Print Group

ISBN: 978 0 9974 6775 8

Printed and bound in China

Always do the warm-up exercises before attempting any individual exercises. It is recommended that you check with your doctor or healthcare professional before commencing any exercise regime. While every care has been taken in the preparation of this material, the publishers and their respective employees or agents will not accept responsibility for injury or damage occasioned to any person as a result of participation in the activities described in this book.

Contents

Understanding Your Core

This powerful group of muscles seems to have taken center stage in the world of fitness—and rightfully so.

Today's fitness enthusiasts invoke the term *core* so often that it can be hard to tell what the word really means. It is used in myriad ways—by everyone from the new mother wanting to firm her midsection to the weekend tennis warrior seeking more power in his backhand swing or the sedentary executive just looking to get through the day without lower-back pain. And for anyone who wants improved posture or simply to look slimmer and fitter, the idea of "working the core" holds great currency.

What is the core?

The core comprises a system of muscles in the lower trunk area including the lower back, abdomen, and hips. These muscles work together to provide support and mobility, and it is in them that all bodily movement, in every conceivable direction, originates.

The major core muscles include the abdominals, the spinal extensors, and the hip flexors and extensors. The abdominal muscles, or the "abs," consist of the rectus abdominis, transversus abdominis, and the internal and external obliques. The rectus abdominis, commonly called the "six-pack," is responsible for maintaining spine stability as well as shortening the distance between your torso and hips. The transversus abdominis provides thoracic and pelvic stability. Both the internal and external obliques are responsible for your ability to bend from side to side and rotate your torso. The Christmas tree-shaped erector spinae is actually a group of muscles and tendons that stretches from the lumbar to the cervical spine. The erector spinae is responsible for stabilization as well as movement of your spine. The hip flexors (iliopsoas, iliacus, rectus femoris, sartorius, tensor fasciae latae, pectineus, adductor longus, adductor brevis, and gracilis) and hip extensors (gluteus maximus, biceps femoris, semitendinosus, and semimembranosus) act as the basement of this muscular powerhouse, supporting movement and allowing you to flex and extend your hips.

A strong core is paramount to keeping the body functionally sound and operational. Many quick-fix diets, pieces of exercise equipment, and even surgeries promise a sleeker, better-looking abdominal area, but it is through core training that focuses on strength and flexibility—coupled with a healthy diet—that real, long-lasting results can come about.

Everyday benefits

Aside from the obvious aesthetic benefits of maintaining a lean and tight core, there are real-world pluses. Imagine easing back pain, standing up straighter (and in the process, looking taller), and being able to move heavy objects without stress or strain. Performing everyday movements becomes easier, even with age. Core training is an insurance policy for keeping the body functional.

Maintaining a strong core will lend optimal support to ancillary (assisting) muscles. In fact, the core is so central to your body's movement that it is called upon whenever any muscle in the body is used. The core

constantly assists other muscle groups, acting as the fulcrum for all motion. For example, lifting an object overhead mainly recruits your deltoids and triceps, but your core muscles also work to both support and balance you, keeping your torso steady as you lift. If your core were not present and firing, it would make proper trunk alignment nearly impossible. That kind of motion, unassisted by the core, would be both much more difficult and potentially dangerous due to spinal compression.

The core is the only muscle system in the body that we train for compactness, rather than for volume as we tend to do with chest muscles. As we train our cores, the ultimate goal is not only to have a sleek, great-looking midsection, but also to attain a functionally sound core that can rotate, contract, and support us in all areas of life.

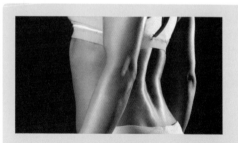

Stronger core = stronger body
Our widespread dependence on artificial support, such as chair backings that shoulder the work of sitting up straight for us, has left many of us soft around the middle. Imagine all of those hours spent slouching, without challenging the core, until upon rising the back feels strained to the point where pain prevails. If you have a sedentary job, you are likely to benefit greatly from challenging your core.

Getting Fit at Home

Core training doesn't have to be expensive. Anyone can follow an effective workout in the privacy of home.

Don't think that you need a huge, intimidating health club with all the latest equipment and extras in order to cultivate an attention-grabbing physique. In truth, some of the fittest bodies have been sculpted in not only less-than-desirable gyms but even in the home with some basic equipment, the desire to improve, and a plan. In fact, a targeted fitness plan performed at home can prove superior to a schedule at a commercial health club that includes a daunting array of high-tech machinery and filled-up classes. At home, you can focus without distractions and at your own pace, experimenting as you see fit in order to keep your workouts interesting.

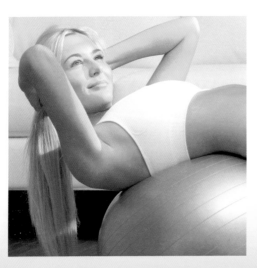

Home-gym equipment

You need very little equipment for effective at-home core training—your own body weight is your best asset, providing resistance. To add variety to your workout, take advantage of objects around the house: chairs can be used for dips and push-ups, while steps can accommodate lunges. Broomsticks come in handy for balancing exercises and twisting movements. If you don't have a mat, a large, thick towel or carpeting will provide light cushioning and prevent you from sliding on the floor.

Your workout wardrobe

Think comfort, utility, and yes, style when deciding what to wear for your workout. Invest in sneakers or trainers with good cushioning and support; your feet are your foundation.

Dress for breathability, insulation, and functional comfort, choosing garments that allow you to move freely. This doesn't mean that you should throw on shapeless T-shirts or baggy sweatpants; form-fitting shorts and tops move with your natural musculature rather than restricting it. Exercise in front of a mirror whenever possible, too. At the start of your workout plan, you may not like how you look in body-hugging garments, but as you stick to your plan, you'll see the changes to your shape even more clearly. Now *that's* motivation!

A time and place for fitness

Effective exercise begins with setting aside a time and a place. This is your chance to give back to your body and maintain the machine that is you. To get the most out of your effort, the location should be free of distractions and allow for clear focus on the task at hand. Elements like music, room temperature, and lighting all have an effect on ensuring the best possible workout. A great thing about working out at home is that you can keep these elements personalized to your own taste.

Make sure that your workout surface is comfortable. If you are exercising on a mat, roll it out properly, ensuring that it is flat, with no loose ends curling upward.

Leave plenty of space around the mat. It is important that you can freely elongate your muscles; incomplete extensions can lead to incomplete muscular development. A full range of motion is vital to your progress.

Now that you are set to begin your workout, you must be present. This may seem like a no-brainer at first, but in today's ultra-fast-paced world, it is easy to become distracted by what you think you may be missing while working out. Try to leave all of your concerns outside your workout space; the world will still exist in all its complexity once your session is over.

For many, making time and space to take care of the body is the hardest part; simply getting ready to exercise, whether this involves going to the gym or setting up a mat at home, takes discipline, time management, and commitment. Now, make the most of it by bettering you.

Fitness balls
A low-tech extra like the antiburst fitness ball shown in several of the following exercises will add another dimension to your at-home routine. This heavy-duty inflatable ball—known by many names, including Swiss ball, exercise ball, body ball, and balance ball—was originally developed for use by physical therapy patients, but it is now standard equipment in commercial and home gyms everywhere. Working on a fitness ball, which ranges in size from 14 to 34 inches (35–85 cm), calls for you to constantly adjust your balance, which forces the engagement of many more muscles, especially those of your core. You can perform both core-stabilizing and core-strengthening exercises on a fitness ball.

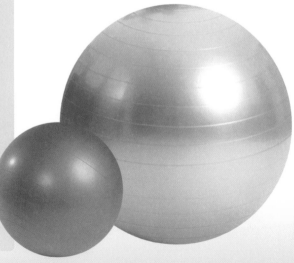

Core Training Basics

Most weight-resistance programs target specific muscle groups, but core training is about treating the body as a unified whole. Although you may feel some of the exercises in this book in one region of your body more strongly than in others, these core workouts are designed to improve muscular function, strengthening, and stabilization throughout your entire body.

You draw upon your core muscles every single day. Although rarely in daily life will you find yourself contracting your biceps or extending your arms to full lockout from your chest as if you're doing a bench press, it's not uncommon to lift an object off the ground and rotate your trunk in order to put it down. This movement is accomplished through reliance on not one isolated muscle, but rather on a group of muscles, including the core, working together.

Breathing, speed, and form are key when working the core. With a firm command of these three elements, you can develop your core muscles efficiently and effectively. Endless repetitions are neither necessary nor advisable; you need only carry out a few calculated sets to achieve a deep muscular burn.

Your breathing pace should be natural and steady. Couple a deep inhale with the negative, or stretching, of the muscle. Think of the inhalation as pulling back the arrow on a bow before launch, and follow it with a deep exhale on the positive, or extended, portion of the movement, as if you were releasing the arrow. Aim for a slow or controlled negative followed by an explosive positive and a slight hold at the peak contraction or finished position. Neither rush through your reps nor greatly slow them; instead, adopt a natural pace that you can sustain throughout the set.

For best results, give your all during each and every rep performed. That guy who claims that he can do a thousand sit-ups would in reality be lucky to complete a hundred that truly work his core, because the neck and lower back—not to mention speed and momentum—are usually called into play when so many repetitions are involved. For best results, less is more: aim to lengthen the muscle, then contract and squeeze. Place the tension on the core muscles at hand without calling in recruits.

Warming up

The following pages include two warm-up stretches followed by both core-stabilizing and core-strengthening exercises. Warm-ups are essential components of a successful fitness regime. You should perform two kinds: cardiovascular exercises and stretches. Jumping rope, boxing, running, cycling—any sustained exertion that gets your heart pumping—will get blood and oxygen moving through your body. Stretches will improve your flexibility, which in turn decreases your risk of injury.

Core stability

Core-stabilizing exercises help to support your core during motion. To stabilize is to both secure your spine and work your visible abdominal muscles. During the execution of a core-stabilizing exercise, your spine should remain in a neutral position without any movement.

Stability exercises focus on improving your core functionality over defining your abdominal musculature.

Core strength

Core-strengthening exercises work the core directly, building strength and endurance as well as muscles. These are the moves that can give you the "six-pack" abs look, in which each segment of the rectus abdominis is highly defined.

Core-strengthening exercises generally target the rectus abdominis, transversus abdominis, and obliques. In the process, the muscles of the midsection become more compact.

Nutrition for core training

When we train our cores, we are aiming for a physique that is both low in visible body fat and high in lean muscle tissue—a physique most definitely achievable. You can maintain a fit core over the long term by carrying out a solid day-to-day plan that combines stretching and strengthening exercises with sound food choices.

For best results, you must fuel properly. The old adage that you are what you eat applies quite literally to the physique. Almost anyone can achieve a "thin" or even "skinny" state by severely limiting food intake, but relying on a drastic reduction of calories often comes at the expense of precious muscle tissue. And a starvation diet usually results in a rebound effect, with the overzealous dieter soon gaining back all of the lost weight and then some.

When it comes to fat loss, the most common mistake lies in overtraining, and in the process breaking the body down to the point of lethargy and exhaustion, while also failing to eat enough to power the body. Too many of us skip breakfast or depend on a last-minute stimulant like coffee—which may fuel us through a few hours—but burnout is inevitable. For optimal results, consume small, frequent meals throughout the day in order to keep your body energized, sparing muscle and instead utilizing stored fat as fuel.

The kinds of food that make up an ideal diet can be divided into three groups: proteins, which help to build muscle mass; fats, which are good for joint lubrication, maintaining body temperature, and promoting healthy cell function in our hair and skin; and carbohydrates, which provide energy.

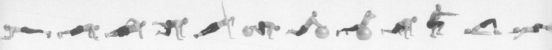

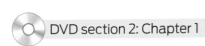

Half-Kneeling Rotation

Warming up is essential before any workout. The following two exercises will improve your flexibility. Half-Kneeling Rotation is a warm-up stretch that increases your spinal mobility, improves your posture, and enhances your core rotation.

1 Kneel on one leg with your right leg bent at 90 degrees in front of you, foot on the floor. Your hands should be beside your head and your elbows should be flared outward.

2 Keeping your back straight, rotate your left shoulder toward your right knee. Hold for 10 seconds, and then repeat on the other side. Work up to 10 repetitions per side.

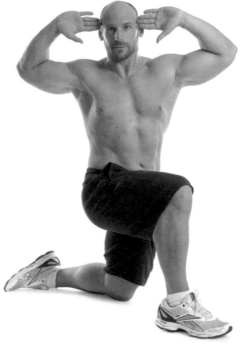

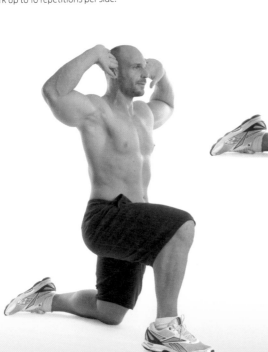

Correct form
· Keep your back straight.

Avoid
· Overextension.

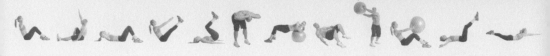

Diary of practice

	Date	Repetitions	Comment
Week 1			
Week 2			
Week 3			
Week 4			

 DVD section 2: Chapter 2

Supine Lower-Back Stretch

Supine Lower-Back Stretch is an excellent warm-up that stretches your lower-back and gluteal muscles.

1 Lie on your back, with legs bent and hands clasped around your knees.

2 Slowly pull your knees toward your chest until you feel a stretch in your lower back.

3 Hold for 30 seconds, relax, and repeat for an additional 30 seconds.

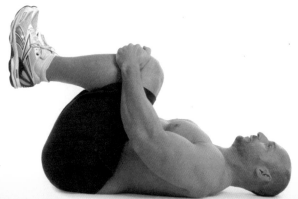

Correct form
· Keep your knees and feet together.

Avoid
· Raising your head off the floor.

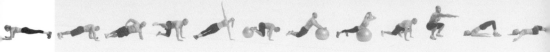

Plank

Plank is an isometric, or contracted, core-stabilizing exercise, designed to work your entire core. It is performed everywhere from yoga and Pilates studios to hard-core gyms for a good reason: it is a reliable way to build endurance in your abs and back, as well as the stabilizer muscles.

1 Begin on an exercise mat on your hands and knees in a facedown position.

2 Plant your forearms on the floor, parallel to each other.

3 Raise your knees off the floor and lengthen your legs until they are in line with your arms. Remain suspended in Plank for 30 seconds, building up to 2 minutes.

Correct form
- Keep your abdominal muscles tight.
- Keep your body in a straight line.

Avoid
- Bridging too high, which can take stress off working muscles.

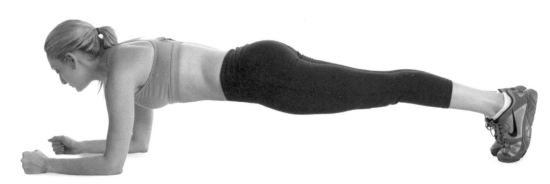

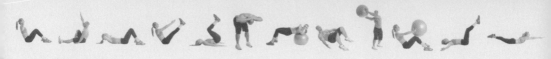

Diary of practice

	Date	Time held	Comment
Week 1			
Week 2			
Week 3			
Week 4			

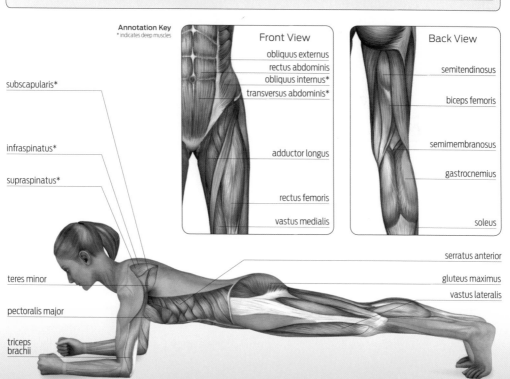

Annotation Key
* indicates deep muscles

Front View
obliquus externus
rectus abdominis
obliquus internus*
transversus abdominis*

adductor longus

rectus femoris

vastus medialis

Back View
semitendinosus

biceps femoris

semimembranosus

gastrocnemius

soleus

subscapularis*

infraspinatus*

supraspinatus*

teres minor

pectoralis major

triceps brachii

serratus anterior

gluteus maximus

vastus lateralis

Plank-Up

Plank-Up is an advanced core-stabilizing exercise that expands upon the basic Plank exercise. Try to maintain a steady rhythm.

1 Begin on your hands and knees in a facedown position. Plant your forearms on the floor parallel to each other.

2 Raise your knees off the floor and lengthen your legs until they are in line with your arms.

3 Lift up with your right arm until it is fully extended, and then straighten your left arm until you are balanced on both arms in a completed push-up position.

4 Reverse one arm at a time, lowering from the planted hand to forearm until back in the initial plank position. Begin with 10 complete repetitions and work up to 2 sets of 15.

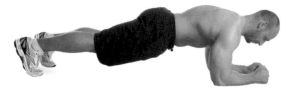

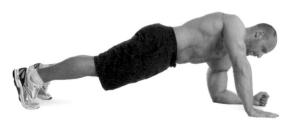

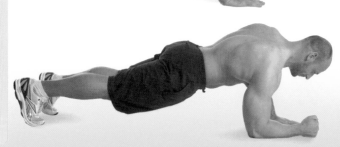

Correct form
· Plant each hand, rather than using momentum, which places too much stress on the joints.
· Keep your abs tucked tightly during the movement.

Avoid
· Crashing down suddenly. Instead, use a steady 4-count motion: 2 up for both arms, then 2 down.

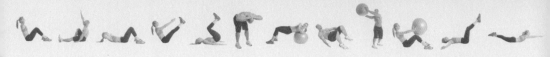

Diary of practice

	Date	Repetitions	Comment
Week 1			
Week 2			
Week 3			
Week 4			

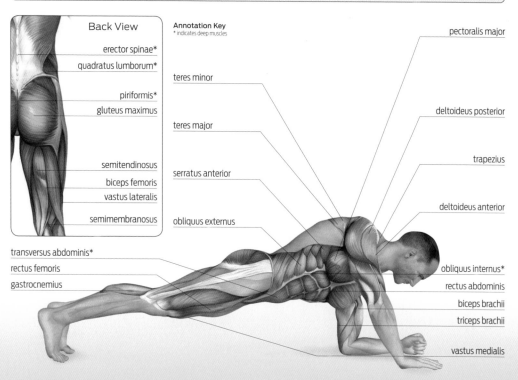

Back View

erector spinae*
quadratus lumborum*
piriformis*
gluteus maximus
semitendinosus
biceps femoris
vastus lateralis
semimembranosus

Annotation Key
* indicates deep muscles

teres minor
teres major
serratus anterior
obliquus externus

transversus abdominis*
rectus femoris
gastrocnemius

pectoralis major
deltoideus posterior
trapezius
deltoideus anterior
obliquus internus*
rectus abdominis
biceps brachii
triceps brachii
vastus medialis

 DVD section 2: Chapter 5

Side Plank

Side Plank stabilizes your spine, but it is also great for strengthening your abdominals, lower back, and shoulders.

1 Lie on your left side with your legs straight and parallel to each other. Keep your feet flexed.

2 Bend your left arm to a 90-degree angle with the knuckles of your hand facing forward. Place your right hand on your waist or extend your arm along your side.

3 Pressing your forearm down into the floor, raise your hips until your body is in a straight line. Hold for 30 seconds, working up to 1 minute. Repeat on the other side.

Correct form
· Push evenly from both your forearm and hips.

Avoid
· Placing too much strain on your shoulders; they should neither sink into their sockets nor lift toward your ears.

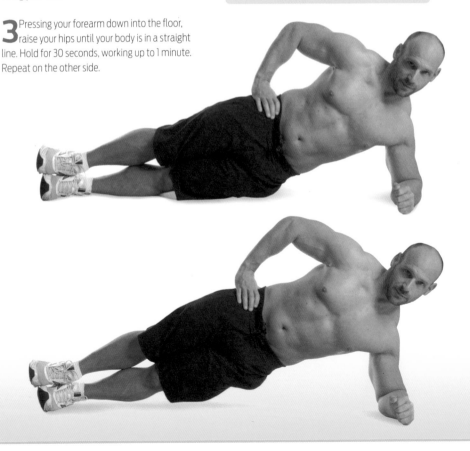

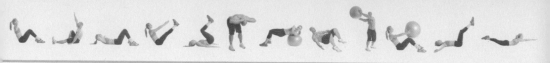

Diary of practice

	Date	Time held	Comment
Week 1			
Week 2			
Week 3			
Week 4			

Annotation Key
* indicates deep muscles

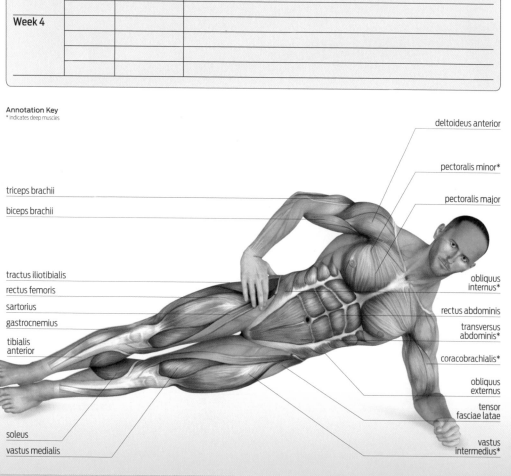

triceps brachii

biceps brachii

tractus iliotibialis

rectus femoris

sartorius

gastrocnemius

tibialis anterior

soleus

vastus medialis

deltoideus anterior

pectoralis minor*

pectoralis major

obliquus internus*

rectus abdominis

transversus abdominis*

coracobrachialis*

obliquus externus

tensor fasciae latae

vastus intermedius*

Fire Hydrant In-Out

Fire Hydrant In-Out is a hard-working core-stabilizing exercise, as well as a great core-strengthener. It targets your inner thighs, hamstrings, and glutes, with assistance from your abdominal muscles.

1 Begin on your hands and knees, with your palms on the floor and spaced shoulder-width apart. Your spine should be in a neutral position.

2 Keeping your right leg bent at a 90-degree angle, raise it laterally, or to the side.

3 Straighten your right leg until it is fully extended behind you so that it is in line with your torso.

4 Bend your right knee and bring your leg back into its 90-degree position, and then lower it to meet your left leg. Work up to 15 repetitions. Repeat on the other side.

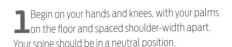

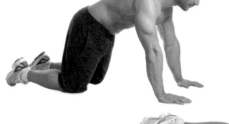

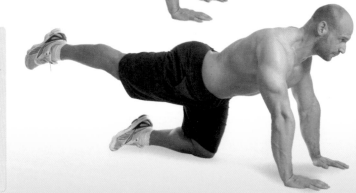

Correct form
- Press your hands into the floor to keep your shoulders from sinking.
- Squeeze your gluteal muscles with your leg fully extended.

Avoid
- Lifting your hip as you lift your bent leg to the side.
- Rushing through the exercise; make sure that you feel each portion of the repetition.

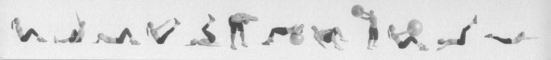

Diary of practice

	Date	Repetitions	Comment
Week 1			
Week 2			
Week 3			
Week 4			

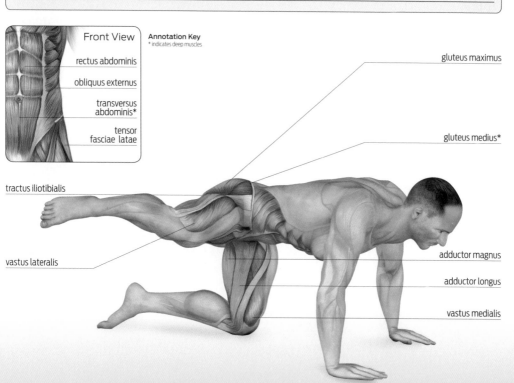

Front View

Annotation Key
* indicates deep muscles

rectus abdominis
obliquus externus
transversus abdominis*
tensor fasciae latae

tractus iliotibialis

vastus lateralis

gluteus maximus

gluteus medius*

adductor magnus

adductor longus

vastus medialis

 DVD section 2: Chapter 7

T-Stabilization

T-Stabilization, another advanced variation on the traditional Plank, is a proven exercise for targeting your abs, hips, lower back, and obliques.

1 Assume the finished push-up position with your arms extended to full lockout, your fingers facing forward, your legs outstretched, and your body weight supported on your toes.

2 Turn your hips to one side, collapsing one foot on top of the other and raising your top arm across your body until you are pointing toward the ceiling.

3 Hold for 30 seconds, lower, and then repeat on the other side. Work your way up to holding for 1 minute on each side.

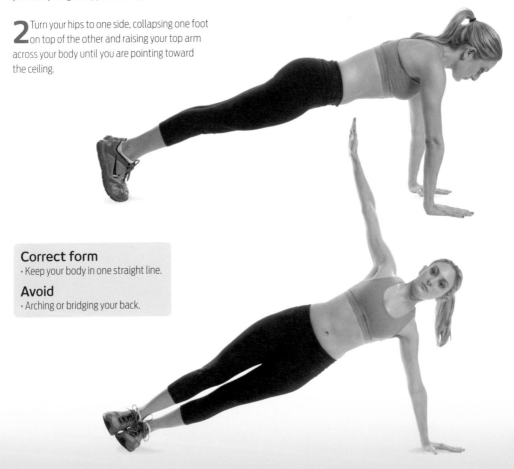

Correct form
· Keep your body in one straight line.

Avoid
· Arching or bridging your back.

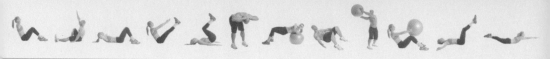

Diary of practice

	Date	Time held	Comment
Week 1			
Week 2			
Week 3			
Week 4			

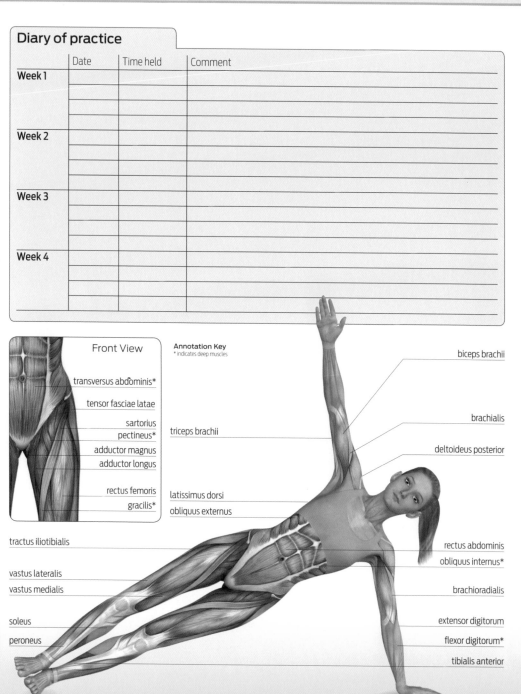

Front View

Annotation Key
* indicates deep muscles

transversus abdominis*
tensor fasciae latae
sartorius
pectineus*
adductor magnus
adductor longus
rectus femoris
gracilis*

triceps brachii

latissimus dorsi
obliquus externus

tractus iliotibialis

vastus lateralis
vastus medialis

soleus
peroneus

biceps brachii

brachialis

deltoideus posterior

rectus abdominis
obliquus internus*

brachioradialis

extensor digitorum
flexor digitorum*

tibialis anterior

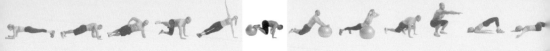

Fitness Ball Atomic Push-Up

Performing the Fitness Ball Atomic Push-Up causes many major muscle groups to fire at once. When executed properly, this exercise tones your upper body, engages your core, and works your hip flexors.

1 Begin on your hands and knees with your fingers facing forward and a fitness ball placed behind you. Rest your shins on the ball, and straighten your legs so that your body forms a straight line.

2 While keeping your back flat, bend your knees to draw the fitness ball into your core.

3 Straighten your legs, moving the ball farther behind you, and then perform a push-up. Start with 5 repetitions, working your way up to 2 sets of 12 to 15.

Correct form
· Keep your hips level with your torso.

Avoid
· Piking or bridging your body.

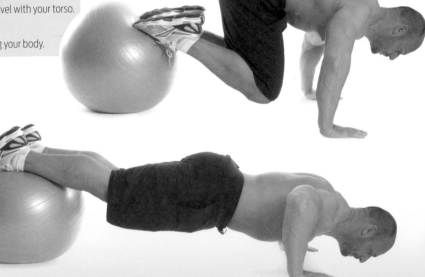

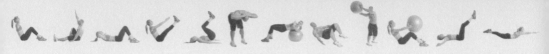

Diary of practice

	Date	Repetitions	Comment
Week 1			
Week 2			
Week 3			
Week 4			

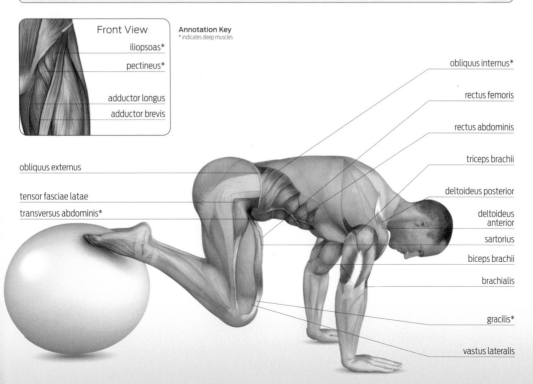

Front View

iliopsoas*

pectineus*

adductor longus

adductor brevis

Annotation Key
* indicates deep muscles

obliquus internus*

rectus femoris

rectus abdominis

triceps brachii

deltoideus posterior

deltoideus anterior

sartorius

biceps brachii

brachialis

gracilis*

vastus lateralis

obliquus externus

tensor fasciae latae

transversus abdominis*

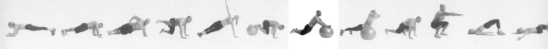

DVD section 2: Chapter 9

Fitness Ball Rollout

Fitness Ball Rollout is a fun and challenging exercise for effectively stabilizing your core. Aim for controlled, steady movement throughout.

1 Kneel behind your fitness ball, with your fists resting on top of it.

2 Extend the ball forward, leading with your arms and following with your body until you are completely stretched out while maintaining a flat back and staying anchored on your knees.

3 Using your abdominals and lower back, roll back in until you reach an upright position. Work up to 3 sets of 15 repetitions.

Correct form
· Keep your body elongated throughout the movement.

Avoid
· Bridging your back and allowing your hips to sag.

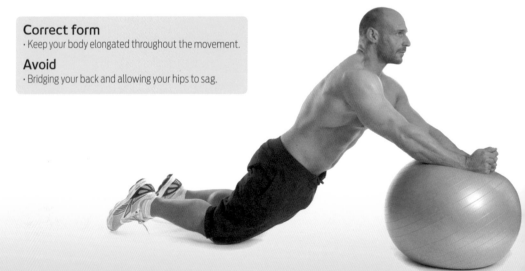

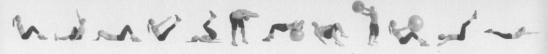

Diary of practice

	Date	Repetitions	Comment
Week 1			
Week 2			
Week 3			
Week 4			

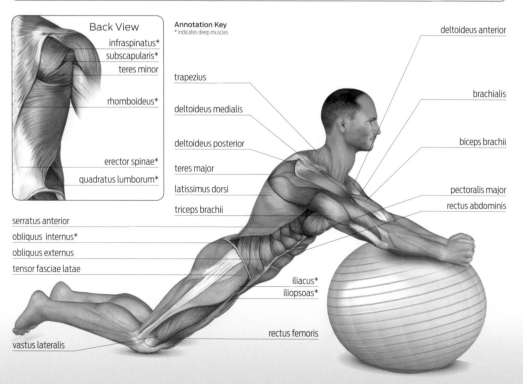

Back View

infraspinatus*
subscapularis*
teres minor

rhomboideus*

erector spinae*
quadratus lumborum*

Annotation Key
* indicates deep muscles

trapezius

deltoideus medialis

deltoideus posterior

teres major

latissimus dorsi

triceps brachii

serratus anterior
obliquus internus*
obliquus externus
tensor fasciae latae

iliacus*
iliopsoas*

rectus femoris

vastus lateralis

deltoideus anterior

brachialis

biceps brachii

pectoralis major
rectus abdominis

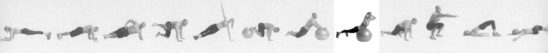

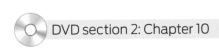

DVD section 2: Chapter 10

Fitness Ball Hyperextension

Fitness Ball Hyperextension, executed on the large fitness ball, is a
safe and effective alternative to traditional hyperextension machines.
Performing this exercise is a great way to work your lower-back muscles.

1 Begin in a facedown position on top of the fitness ball, with your abdominals covering most of the ball, your legs spread with toes on the floor, and your arms behind your head. Push your toes into the floor for stability.

2 Raise your torso so that it forms a line with the lower half of your body.

3 Squeeze your gluteal muscles as you lower your upper body, and then raise it back to the starting position. Continue lowering and raising, working up to 3 sets of 15 to 20 repetitions.

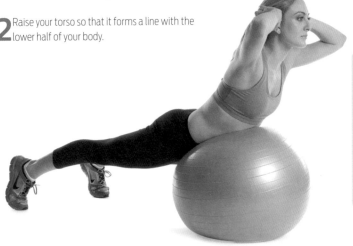

Correct form
- Be sure to complete the full range of motion in both the negative (downward stretch) and positive (upward motion) of the exercise.

Avoid
- Overcontracting or hyperextending your back at the top of the movement.

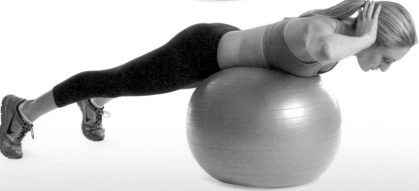

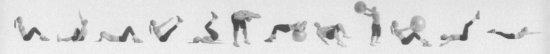

Diary of practice

	Date	Repetitions	Comment
Week 1			
Week 2			
Week 3			
Week 4			

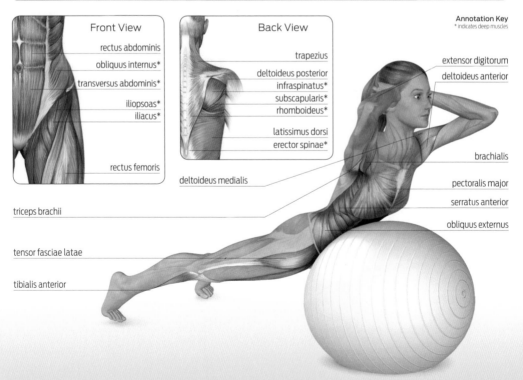

Front View

rectus abdominis
obliquus internus*
transversus abdominis*
iliopsoas*
iliacus*

rectus femoris

triceps brachii

tensor fasciae latae

tibialis anterior

Back View

trapezius
deltoideus posterior
infraspinatus*
subscapularis*
rhomboideus*

latissimus dorsi
erector spinae*

deltoideus medialis

Annotation Key
* indicates deep muscles

extensor digitorum
deltoideus anterior

brachialis

pectoralis major
serratus anterior
obliquus externus

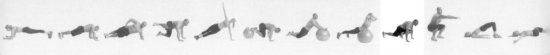

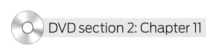
Mountain Climber

Mountain Climber is a core-stabilizing, timed distance exercise. This high-intensity move gets your heart rate going, improving your cardiovascular fitness, while it challenges your legs and core. This all-around exercise also helps to develop muscular endurance in your arms.

1 Begin in a completed push-up position with your body forming a straight line.

2 Bend one knee and bring it as close to your chest as possible.

3 Return to the starting position and repeat with your other leg. Continue to alternate for 30 seconds, working up to 2 minutes.

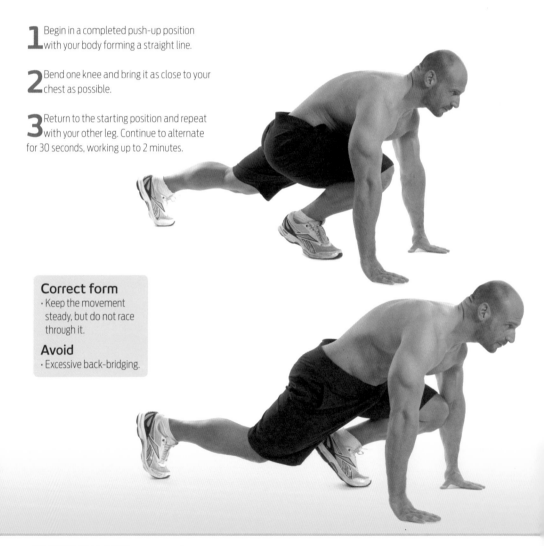

Correct form
· Keep the movement steady, but do not race through it.

Avoid
· Excessive back-bridging.

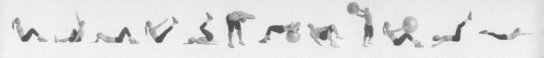

Diary of practice

	Date	Repetitions	Comment
Week 1			
Week 2			
Week 3			
Week 4			

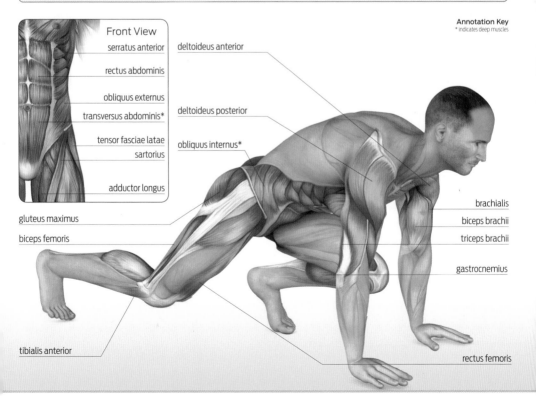

Annotation Key
* indicates deep muscles

Front View

serratus anterior

rectus abdominis

obliquus externus

transversus abdominis*

tensor fasciae latae

sartorius

adductor longus

gluteus maximus

biceps femoris

tibialis anterior

deltoideus anterior

deltoideus posterior

obliquus internus*

brachialis

biceps brachii

triceps brachii

gastrocnemius

rectus femoris

 DVD section 2: Chapter 12

Body-Weight Squat

Body-Weight Squat is a full-body exercise. Completing it correctly means using your core properly. It may look like an easy move, but there is more to it: as well as engaging your leg muscles, it engages nearly every muscle in your lower body. Perfecting this exercise is a great way to combat the weakness that often develops from a sedentary lifestyle.

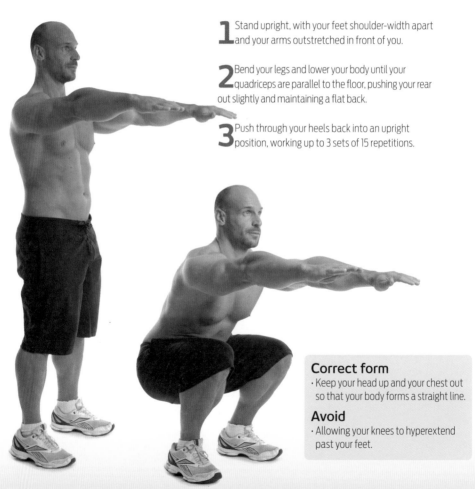

1 Stand upright, with your feet shoulder-width apart and your arms outstretched in front of you.

2 Bend your legs and lower your body until your quadriceps are parallel to the floor, pushing your rear out slightly and maintaining a flat back.

3 Push through your heels back into an upright position, working up to 3 sets of 15 repetitions.

Correct form
· Keep your head up and your chest out so that your body forms a straight line.

Avoid
· Allowing your knees to hyperextend past your feet.

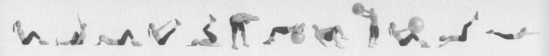

Diary of practice

	Date	Repetitions	Comment
Week 1			
Week 2			
Week 3			
Week 4			

Annotation Key
* indicates deep muscles

obliquus externus

transversus abdominis*

gluteus medius*

tensor fasciae latae

gluteus maximus

biceps femoris

gastrocnemius

sartorius

vastus intermedius*

rectus femoris

vastus medialis

adductor magnus

soleus

tibialis anterior

abductor hallucis

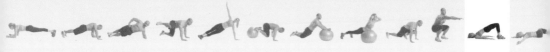

 DVD section 2: Chapter 13

Hip Raise

Adding movement to the traditional Shoulder Bridge, Hip Raise really challenges your core strength. It is not only an abdominal and lower-back exercise, but it also targets your gluteal and hamstring muscles.

1 Lie on your back with your legs bent, your feet flat on the floor, and your arms along your sides.

2 Push through your heels while raising your pelvis until your torso is aligned with your thighs. Lower and then repeat, working up to 3 sets of 15.

Correct form
· Push through your heels, not your toes.

Avoid
· Overextending your abdominals past your thighs in the raised position.

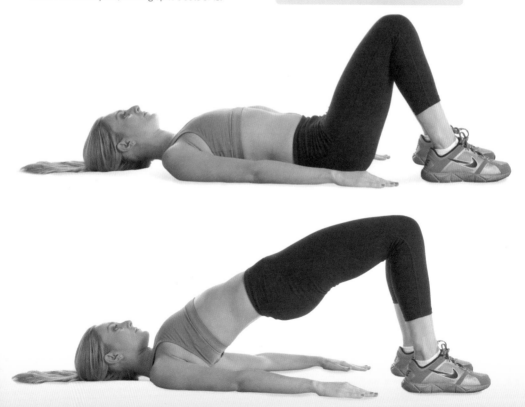

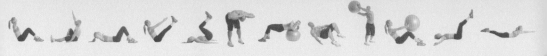

Diary of practice

	Date	Repetitions	Comment
Week 1			
Week 2			
Week 3			
Week 4			

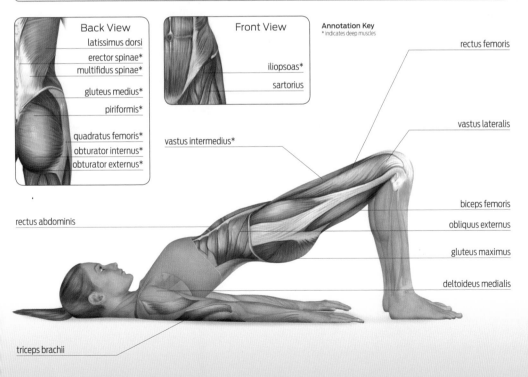

Back View

latissimus dorsi
erector spinae*
multifidus spinae*
gluteus medius*
piriformis*
quadratus femoris*
obturator internus*
obturator externus*

Front View

iliopsoas*
sartorius

Annotation Key
* indicates deep muscles

rectus femoris

vastus lateralis

vastus intermedius*

biceps femoris

obliquus externus

gluteus maximus

deltoideus medialis

rectus abdominis

triceps brachii

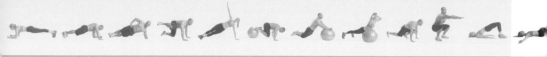

 DVD section 2: Chapter 14

Hip Crossover

Hip Crossover effectively targets your lower-back and oblique muscles. As with many core exercises, when executing Hip Crossover, look for controlled movements. You want your muscles to move you—not momentum.

1 Lie on your back with your arms lengthened away from your body and your legs bent at a 90-degree angle and lifted off the floor.

2 Brace your abs and lower your knees to the side, dropping them as close to the floor as possible without lifting your shoulders off the mat.

3 Return to the starting position, hold for a moment, and then repeat on the other side. Work up to 15 repetitions per side.

Correct form
· Keep your core centered.

Avoid
· Excessively swinging your legs; you want to move carefully and with control.

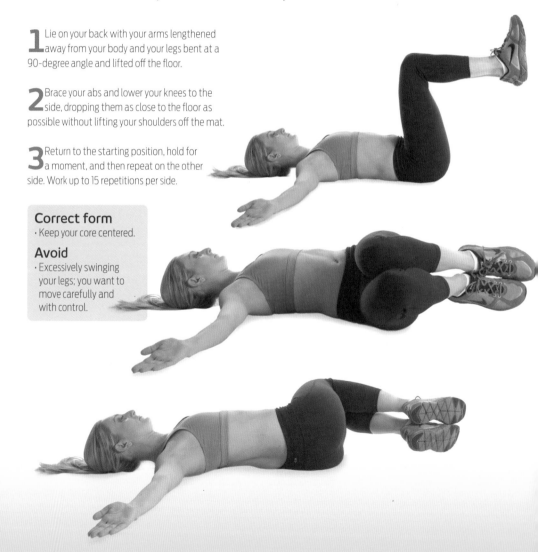

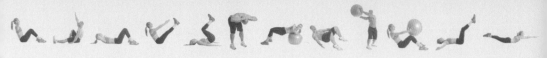

Diary of practice

	Date	Repetitions	Comment
Week 1			
Week 2			
Week 3			
Week 4			

Annotation Key
* indicates deep muscles

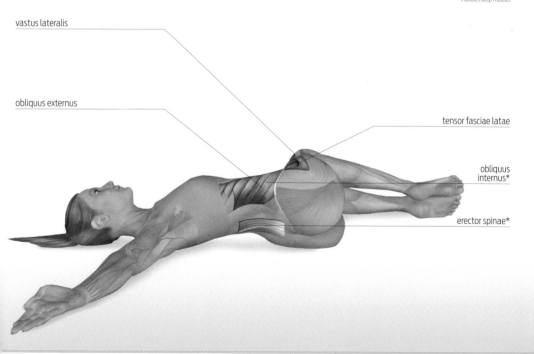

vastus lateralis

obliquus externus

tensor fasciae latae

obliquus internus*

erector spinae*

 DVD section 2: Chapter 15

Sit-Up

The Sit-Up is a basic exercise for both strengthening and defining the abdominal muscles. This workout staple also works the hip flexor muscles. Form is crucial; improperly performed Sit-Ups can strain your spine and the muscles in your head and neck.

1 Lie on your back with your legs bent and your feet firmly planted on the floor. Your hands should be behind your head, your elbows flared outward.

2 Raise your shoulders and torso off the floor toward your legs. Lower and repeat, working up to 3 sets of 20.

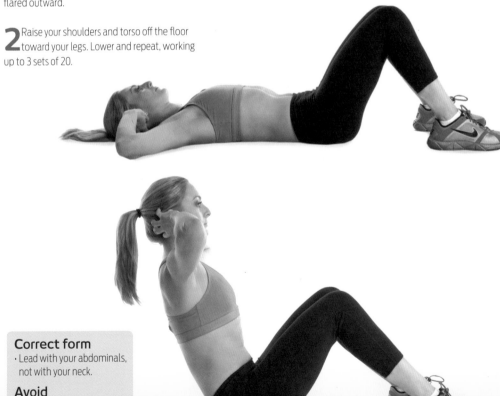

Correct form
· Lead with your abdominals, not with your neck.

Avoid
· Using excessive momentum.
· Overusing your lower back.

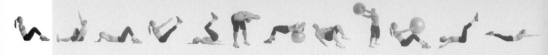

Diary of practice

	Date	Repetitions	Comment
Week 1			
Week 2			
Week 3			
Week 4			

Annotation Key
* indicates deep muscles

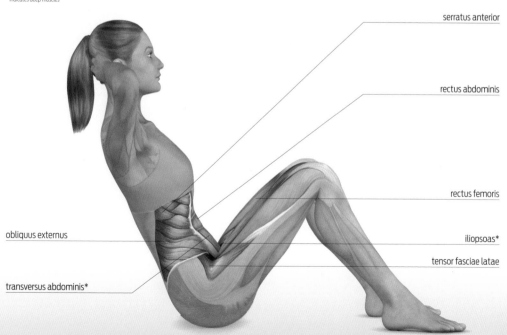

serratus anterior

rectus abdominis

rectus femoris

iliopsoas*

tensor fasciae latae

obliquus externus

transversus abdominis*

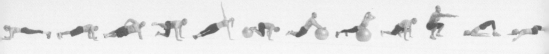

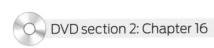
One-Armed Sit-Up

One-Armed Sit-Up is a challenging twist on the traditional Sit-Up, engaging the obliques and the latissimus dorsi, as well as the rectus abdominis.

1 Lie on your back with your left leg bent and your right leg lengthened along the floor. Extend your left arm behind your head, and rest your right arm along your side.

2 Pushing through your left heel, raise your shoulders and torso off the floor until you are sitting nearly upright and your left arm is directly over your head. Lower and repeat on the other side, working up to 2 sets of 15 repetitions.

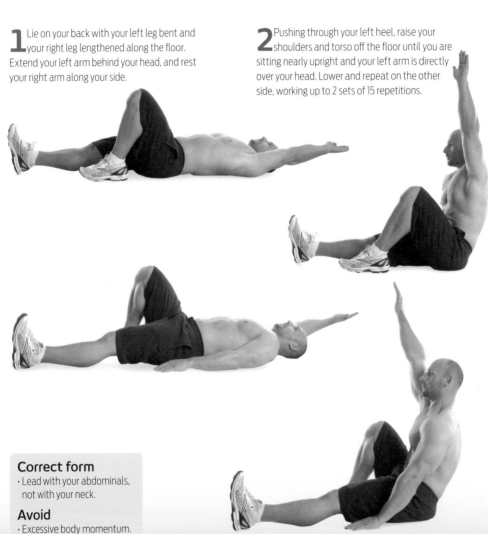

Correct form
· Lead with your abdominals, not with your neck.

Avoid
· Excessive body momentum.
· Overusing your lower back.

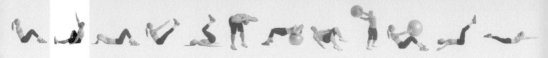

Diary of practice

	Date	Repetitions	Comment
Week 1			
Week 2			
Week 3			
Week 4			

Annotation Key
* indicates deep muscles

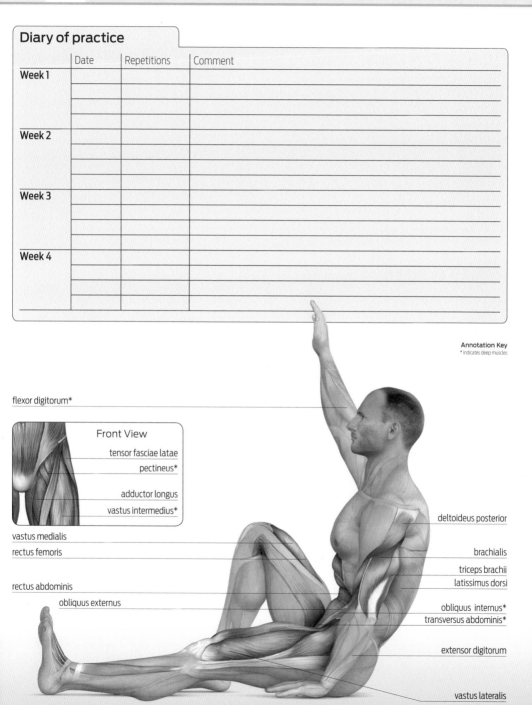

flexor digitorum*

Front View

tensor fasciae latae
pectineus*

adductor longus
vastus intermedius*

vastus medialis
rectus femoris

rectus abdominis
obliquus externus

deltoideus posterior

brachialis
triceps brachii
latissimus dorsi

obliquus internus*
transversus abdominis*

extensor digitorum

vastus lateralis

DVD section 2: Chapter 17

Crunch

Like the Sit-Up, the Crunch is highly effective for isolating the rectus abdominis. Unlike the Sit-Up, however, your lower back never leaves the floor during the movement, which places less strain on the lumbar region of your spine.

1 Lie on your back with your legs bent, elbows flared, and palms next to your ears.

2 Raise your head and shoulders off the floor while contracting your abdominals. Lower and repeat, working up to 3 sets of 25 repetitions.

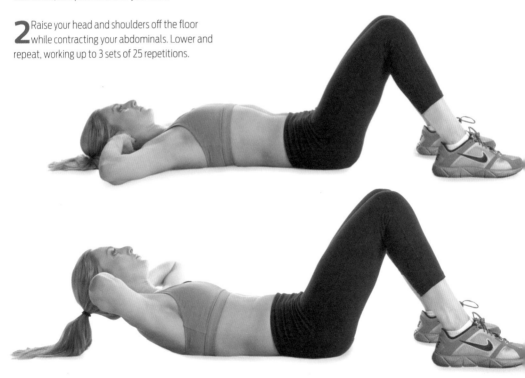

Correct form
· Lead with your abdominals, as if a string were hoisting you up by your belly button.

Avoid
· Overusing your neck.

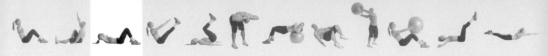

Diary of practice

	Date	Repetitions	Comment
Week 1			
Week 2			
Week 3			
Week 4			

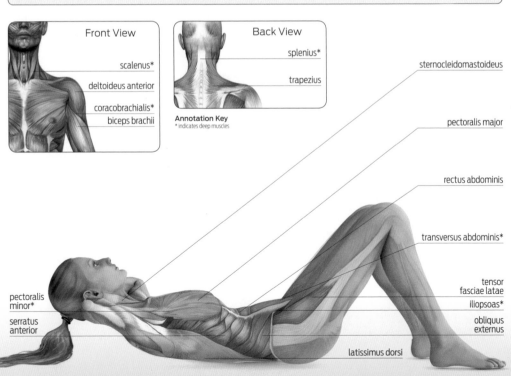

Front View
scalenus*
deltoideus anterior
coracobrachialis*
biceps brachii

Back View
splenius*
trapezius

Annotation Key
* indicates deep muscles

sternocleidomastoideus

pectoralis major

rectus abdominis

transversus abdominis*

tensor fasciae latae

iliopsoas*

obliquus externus

pectoralis minor*

serratus anterior

latissimus dorsi

V-Up

The challenging V-Up targets both your upper and lower rectus abdominis as it moves through its entire range of motion. Performing V-Ups is also an efficient way to strengthen your lower-back muscles and tighten your quads.

1 Lie on your back with your arms and legs elongated on the floor.

2 Simultaneously raise your arms and legs so that your arms are nearly touching your feet, while maintaining a flat back. Lower and repeat, working up to 3 sets of 20 repetitions.

Correct form
· Keep your arms and legs straight.

Avoid
· Using a jerking motion as your raise or lower your arms and legs.

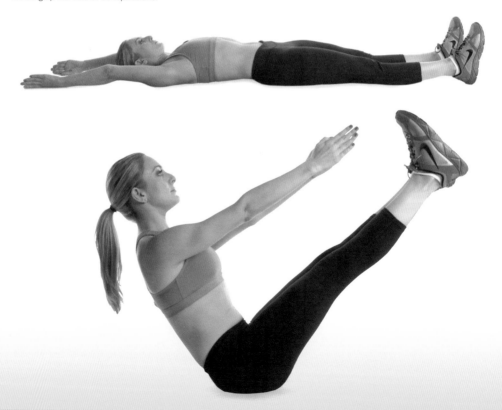

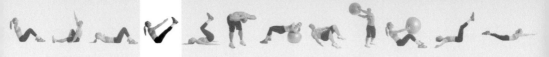

Diary of practice

	Date	Repetitions	Comment
Week 1			
Week 2			
Week 3			
Week 4			

Annotation Key
* indicates deep muscles

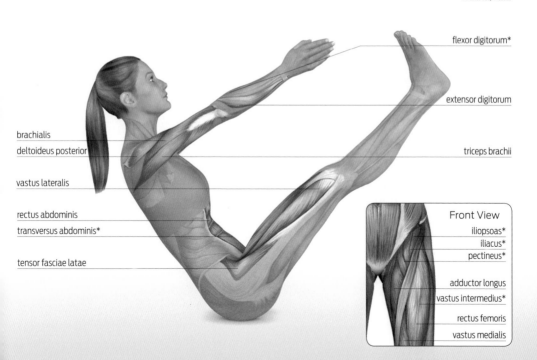

flexor digitorum*

extensor digitorum

brachialis

deltoideus posterior

triceps brachii

vastus lateralis

rectus abdominis

transversus abdominis*

tensor fasciae latae

Front View

iliopsoas*

iliacus*

pectineus*

adductor longus

vastus intermedius*

rectus femoris

vastus medialis

Reverse Crunch

The Reverse Crunch is highly effective for isolating the lowest portion of the rectus abdominis, where most abdominal fat tends to be stored. Less is more with this exercise: your movements should be small but focused.

1 Lie on your back with your arms at your sides and your legs bent at a 90-degree angle with your feet off the floor.

2 Lift your buttocks a few inches off the mat as you bring your knees toward your chest. Lower in a controlled manner. Repeat, working up to 3 sets of 20 repetitions.

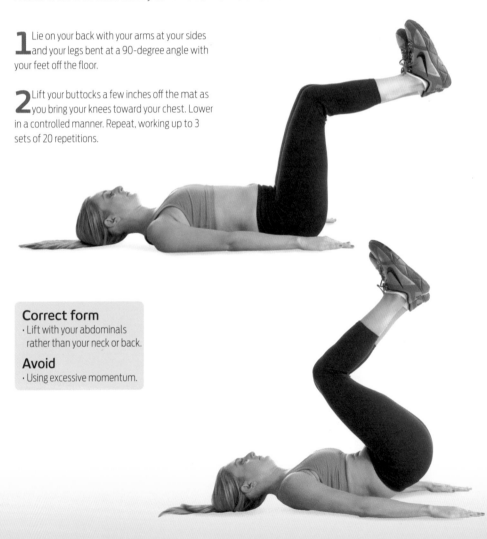

Correct form
· Lift with your abdominals rather than your neck or back.

Avoid
· Using excessive momentum.

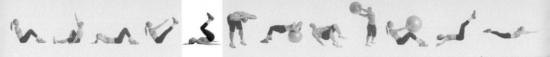

Diary of practice

	Date	Repetitions	Comment
Week 1			
Week 2			
Week 3			
Week 4			

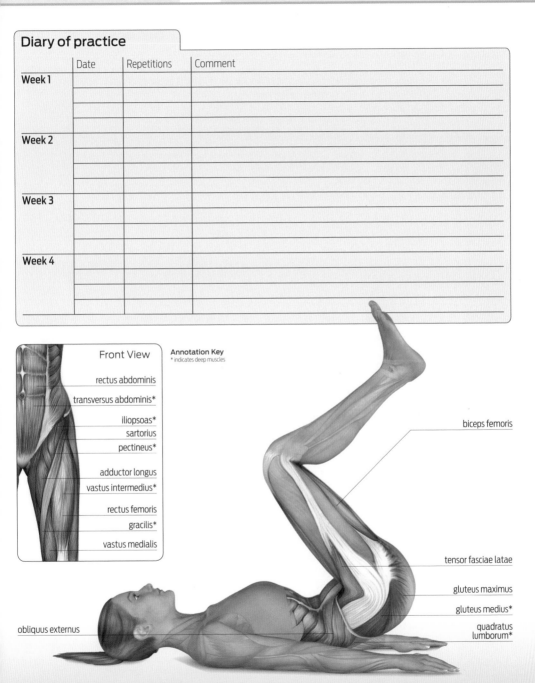

Front View

Annotation Key
* indicates deep muscles

rectus abdominis
transversus abdominis*
iliopsoas*
sartorius
pectineus*
adductor longus
vastus intermedius*
rectus femoris
gracilis*
vastus medialis

obliquus externus

biceps femoris

tensor fasciae latae
gluteus maximus
gluteus medius*
quadratus lumborum*

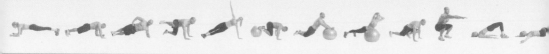

 DVD section 2: Chapter 20

Good Mornings

Good Mornings are effective moves for strengthening your lower back. Weight lifters commonly use a barbell to perform Good Mornings, but here your own body weight provides the resistance for the exercise.

1 Stand upright with your hands clasped behind your head, elbows flared out, and feet shoulder-width apart.

2 Bend your knees slightly and stick your rear out while hinging forward from the waist until your back is nearly parallel to the floor. Return to an upright position and repeat, working up to 3 sets of 15 repetitions.

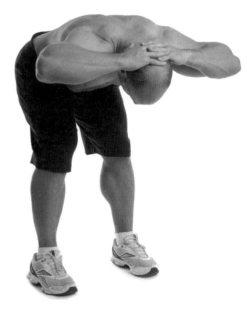

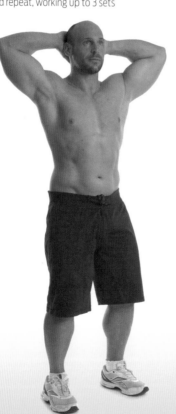

> **Correct form**
> · Perform the exercise slowly and with control.
>
> **Avoid**
> · Rounding your back.

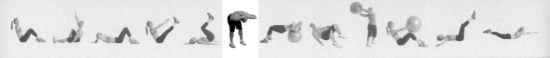

Diary of practice

	Date	Repetitions	Comment
Week 1			
Week 2			
Week 3			
Week 4			

erector spinae*

latissimus dorsi

Annotation Key
* indicates deep muscles

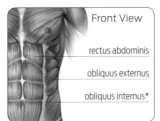

Front View

rectus abdominis

obliquus externus

obliquus internus*

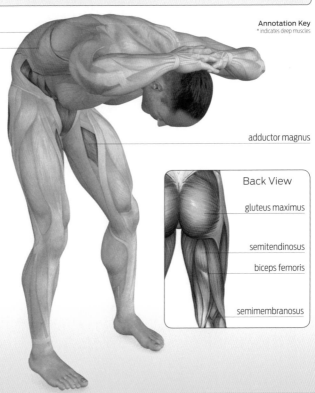

adductor magnus

Back View

gluteus maximus

semitendinosus

biceps femoris

semimembranosus

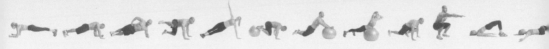

 DVD section 2: Chapter 21

Fitness Ball Russian Twist

Fitness Ball Russian Twist offers a fun, unique way to strengthen your core—and whittle your waistline. It targets all of your abdominals, but because it incorporates rotation, it places an emphasis on the obliques.

1 Sit on your fitness ball, with feet planted shoulder-width apart. Roll forward until your neck is supported on the ball. Extend your arms to full lockout directly above your chest.

2 Turn one hip out to the side while also turning your torso and your arms. Return to the center and repeat on the other side, working up to 3 sets of 15 repetitions per side.

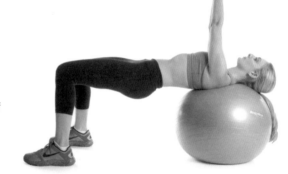

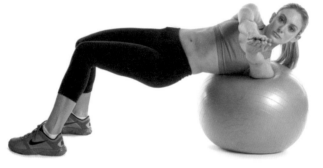

Correct form
· Move slowly and with control.

Avoid
· Allowing your upper back to hang off the fitness ball, unsupported.

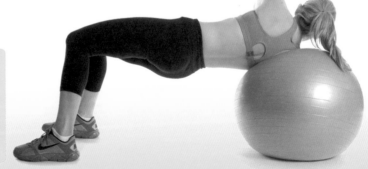

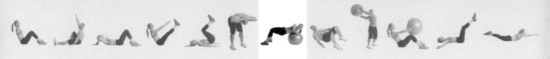

Diary of practice

	Date	Repetitions	Comment
Week 1			
Week 2			
Week 3			
Week 4			

Back View

trapezius

deltoideus medialis

deltoideus posterior

triceps brachii

latissimus dorsi

Front View

deltoideus anterior

biceps brachii

serratus anterior

Annotation Key
* indicates deep muscles

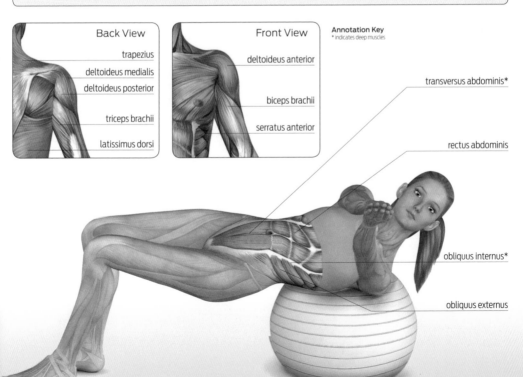

transversus abdominis*

rectus abdominis

obliquus internus*

obliquus externus

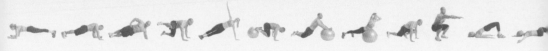

Penguin Crunch

Penguin Crunch, also called the Penguin Heel Reach, targets your oblique muscles. Because it incorporates lateral movement of the abdominals, it is a great exercise to prepare you for any sport that requires rotational movement, such as swimming or diving.

1 Begin on your back, with your head elevated and your arms at your sides and raised off the floor.

2 Reach forward in a stabbing motion with one hand, and then pull back. Lower and repeat with the other hand, working up to 3 sets of 15 repetitions on each side.

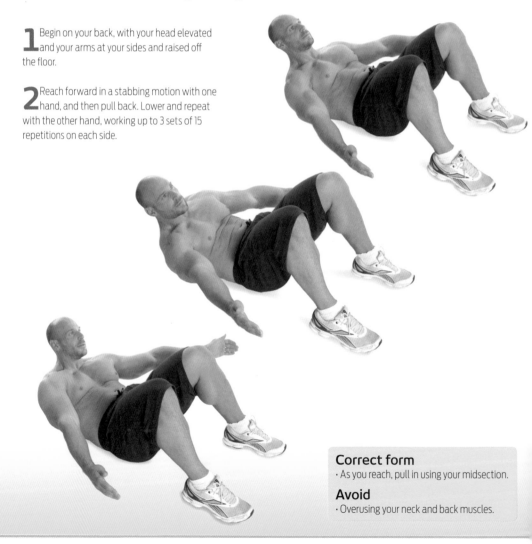

Correct form
· As you reach, pull in using your midsection.

Avoid
· Overusing your neck and back muscles.

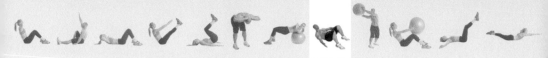

Diary of practice

	Date	Repetitions	Comment
Week 1			
Week 2			
Week 3			
Week 4			

Annotation Key
* indicates deep muscles

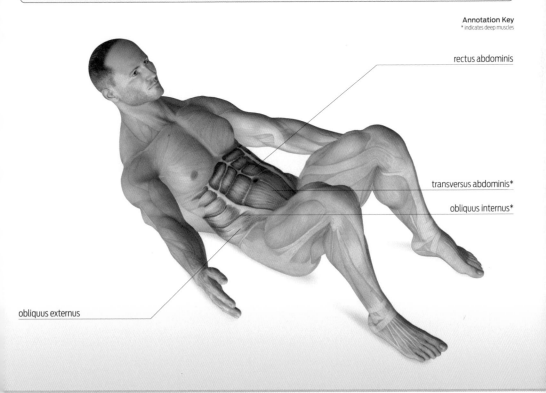

rectus abdominis

transversus abdominis*

obliquus internus*

obliquus externus

 DVD section 2: Chapter 23

Wood Chop with Fitness Ball

Wood Chop with Fitness Ball is another take on a gym classic. Perform this version of the Wood Chop to strengthen your abdominals, especially the oblique muscles. This exercise also works your arm and shoulder muscles.

1 Stand up while holding your large fitness ball. Twist your core to one side, bringing the ball with you.

2 Lower the ball, and then follow through by twisting to the other side and raising it as you turn, as if swinging a baseball bat, while feeling your core contract. Lower the ball. Repeat through the same range of motion on the other side, working up to 3 sets of 20 per side.

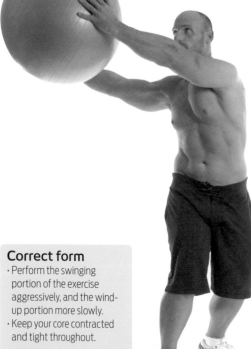

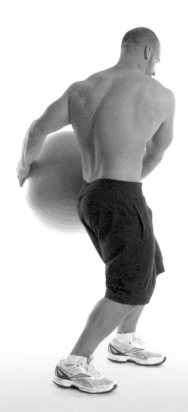

Correct form
- Perform the swinging portion of the exercise aggressively, and the wind-up portion more slowly.
- Keep your core contracted and tight throughout.

Avoid
- Straining your back by twisting too vigorously from side to side.

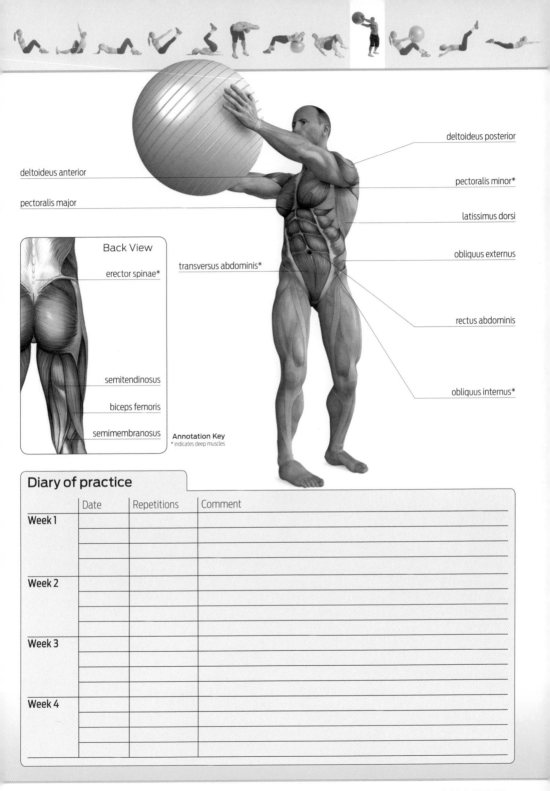

deltoideus posterior

deltoideus anterior

pectoralis minor*

pectoralis major

latissimus dorsi

obliquus externus

Back View

erector spinae*

transversus abdominis*

rectus abdominis

semitendinosus

biceps femoris

obliquus internus*

semimembranosus

Annotation Key
* indicates deep muscles

Diary of practice

	Date	Repetitions	Comment
Week 1			
Week 2			
Week 3			
Week 4			

 DVD section 2: Chapter 24

Fitness Ball Seated Russian Twist

Fitness Ball Seated Russian Twist is effective for strengthening the major muscles of your core, including your obliques, lower-back extensors, abdominals, and deep core stabilizers.

1 Begin seated with your legs apart while holding a fitness ball at arms' length. Lean back slightly to activate your core.

2 While keeping a flat back, begin rotating from side to side. Work up to performing 3 sets of 20 rotations.

Correct form
· Twist with control, and not too speedily.

Avoid
· Rounding your back.

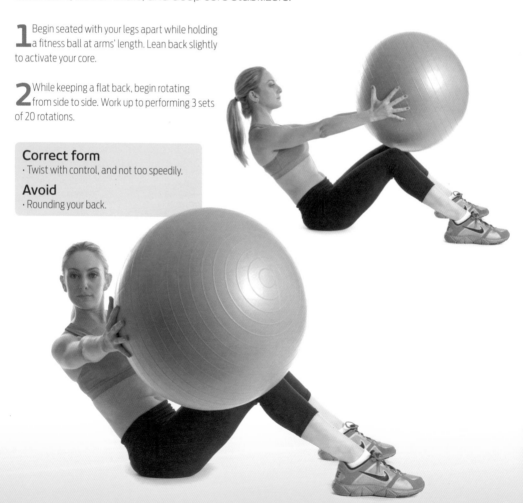

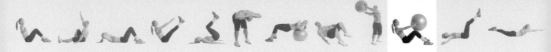

Diary of practice

	Date	Repetitions	Comment
Week 1			
Week 2			
Week 3			
Week 4			

Annotation Key
* indicates deep muscles

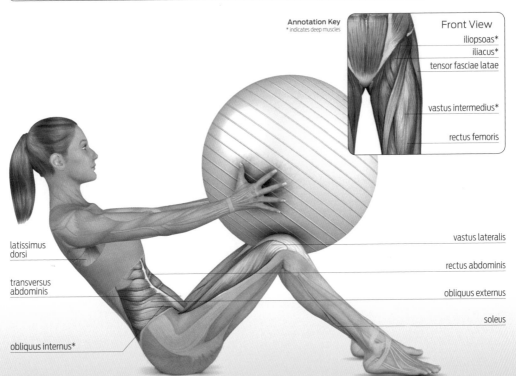

Front View

iliopsoas*
iliacus*
tensor fasciae latae
vastus intermedius*
rectus femoris

latissimus dorsi

transversus abdominis

obliquus internus*

vastus lateralis
rectus abdominis
obliquus externus
soleus

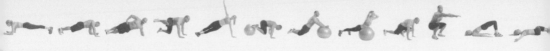

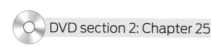

DVD section 2: Chapter 25

Leg Raises

Leg Raises target the transversus abdominis: that tough-to-reach lower abdominal area. This core-strengthening exercise is easy do to, even for most beginners. Perform it regularly to see a reduction in abdominal fat.

1 Lie on your back with your arms out at your sides. Bend your legs slightly and elevate them off the floor.

2 Lower your legs to just above floor level, lift them back up, and repeat. Work up to performing 2 sets of 20 repetitions.

Correct form
· Keep your upper body braced.

Avoid
· Using momentum or your lower back to drive the movement.

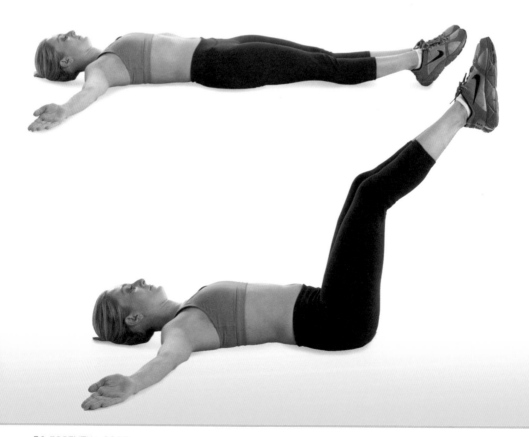

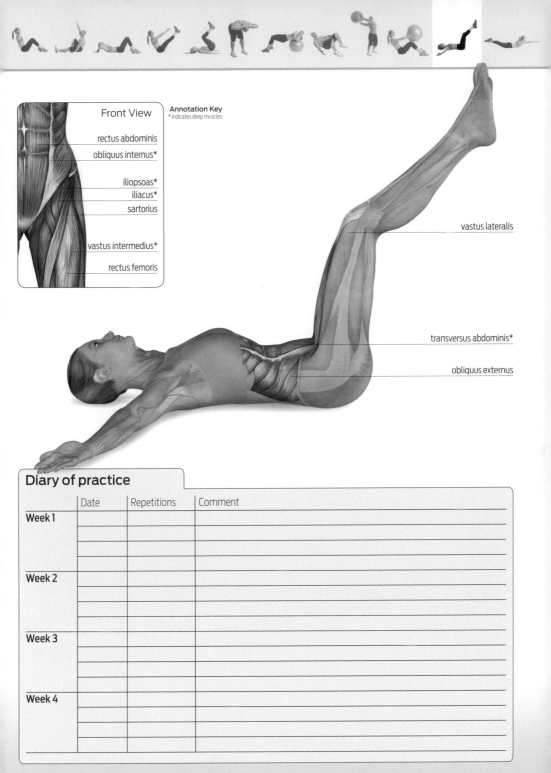

Front View

Annotation Key
* indicates deep muscles

rectus abdominis
obliquus internus*

iliopsoas*
iliacus*
sartorius

vastus intermedius*
rectus femoris

vastus lateralis

transversus abdominis*

obliquus externus

Diary of practice

	Date	Repetitions	Comment
Week 1			
Week 2			
Week 3			
Week 4			

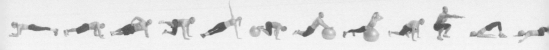

 DVD section 2: Chapter 26

Superman

Superman is great for targeting your entire core as well as your hip flexors and glutes. It is also an effective exercise for your back, strengthening both the full extent of the erector spinae, as well as the multifidus spinae. Beware though—this move is harder than it looks.

1 Lie facedown on your stomach with your arms and legs extended on the floor.

2 Raise your arms and your legs simultaneously, squeezing your glutes at the top, and then lower. Work up to 3 sets of 15.

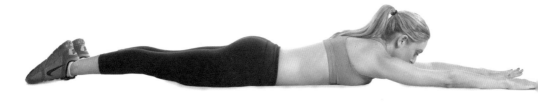

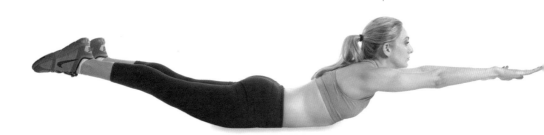

Correct form
· Raise your arms and legs as high as possible.

Avoid
· Overstressing your neck.

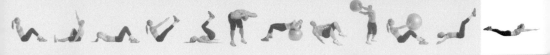

Back View

semitendinosus

vastus lateralis

biceps femoris

semimembranosus

gastrocnemius

Annotation Key
* indicates deep muscles

Back View

semispinalis*

splenius*

trapezius

infraspinatus*

teres minor

teres major

rhomboideus*

latissimus dorsi

erector spinae*

quadratus lumborum*

Front View

sternocleidomastoideus

scalenus*

deltoideus medialis

deltoideus anterior

biceps brachii

flexor digitorum*

extensor
carpi radialis

deltoideus posterior

gluteus maximus

peroneus

tibialis anterior

triceps brachii

rectus femoris

vastus intermedius*

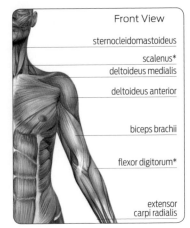

Diary of practice

	Date	Repetitions	Comment
Week 1			
Week 2			
Week 3			
Week 4			

Full-Body Anatomy

scalenus*

pectoralis major

deltoideus anterior

coracobrachialis*

rectus abdominis

obliquus externus

palmaris longus

flexor carpi ulnaris

flexor carpi radialis

transversus abdominis*

sartorius

vastus intermedius*

rectus femoris

vastus lateralis

vastus medialis

tibialis anterior

peroneus

extensor hallucis

adductor hallucis

sternocleidomastoideus

pectoralis minor*

biceps brachii

serratus anterior

obliquus internus*

pronator teres

flexor digitorum*

extensor carpi radialis

flexor carpi pollicis longus

tensor fasciae latae

iliopsoas*

iliacus*

pectineus*

adductor longus

gracilis*

gastrocnemius

soleus

flexor digitorum

extensor digitorum

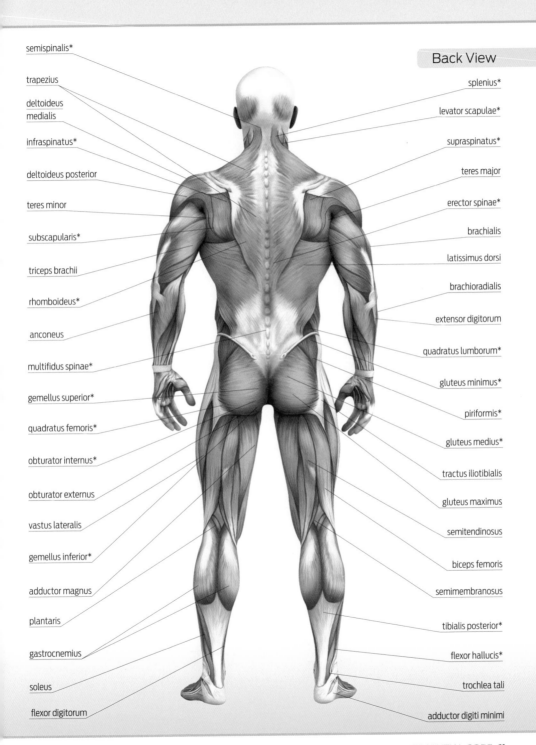

semispinalis*

trapezius

deltoideus
medialis

infraspinatus*

deltoideus posterior

teres minor

subscapularis*

triceps brachii

rhomboideus*

anconeus

multifidus spinae*

gemellus superior*

quadratus femoris*

obturator internus*

obturator externus

vastus lateralis

gemellus inferior*

adductor magnus

plantaris

gastrocnemius

soleus

flexor digitorum

splenius*

levator scapulae*

supraspinatus*

teres major

erector spinae*

brachialis

latissimus dorsi

brachioradialis

extensor digitorum

quadratus lumborum*

gluteus minimus*

piriformis*

gluteus medius*

tractus iliotibialis

gluteus maximus

semitendinosus

biceps femoris

semimembranosus

tibialis posterior*

flexor hallucis*

trochlea tali

adductor digiti minimi

Targeted Workouts

Beginner's Workout
Suitable for all levels, this workout is great for beginners new to core training.

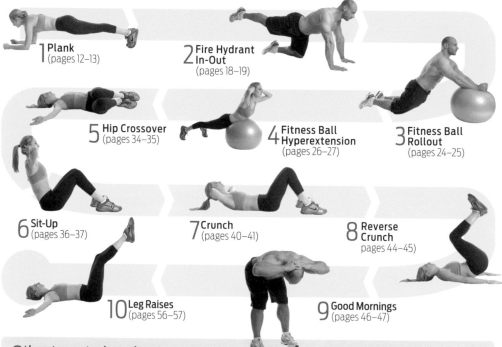

1 **Plank**
(pages 12–13)

2 **Fire Hydrant In-Out**
(pages 18–19)

3 **Fitness Ball Rollout**
(pages 24–25)

4 **Fitness Ball Hyperextension**
(pages 26–27)

5 **Hip Crossover**
(pages 34–35)

6 **Sit-Up**
(pages 36–37)

7 **Crunch**
(pages 40–41)

8 **Reverse Crunch**
pages 44–45)

9 **Good Mornings**
(pages 46–47)

10 **Leg Raises**
(pages 56–57)

Other targeted workouts

Upper-Abdominal Workout
Strengthens and defines your upper abs.
· **Plank-Up** (pages 14–15)
· **T-Stabilization** (pages 20–21)
· **Mountain Climber** (pages 28–29)
· **Sit-Up** (pages 36–37)
· **One-Armed Sit-Up** (pages 38–39)
· **Crunch** (pages 40–41)
· **V-Up** (pages 42–43)
· **Penguin Crunch** (pages 50–51)
· **Wood Chop with Fitness Ball**
  (pages 52–53)
· **Fitness Ball Seated Russian Twist**
  (pages 54–55)

Lower-Abdominal Workout
Strengthens and defines your lower abs.
· **Side Plank** (pages 16–17)
· **Fire Hydrant In-Out** (pages 18–19)
· **T-Stabilization** (pages 20–21)

· **Hip Crossover** (pages 34–35)
· **Hip Raise** (pages 32–33)
· **Reverse Crunch** (pages 44–45)
· **Good Mornings** (pages 46–47)
· **Leg Raise** (pages 56–57)
· **Superman** (pages 58–59)
· **Fitness Ball Russian Twist**
  (pages 48–49)

Global Workout
Incorporates core stabilization and core strengthening for maximum efficiency.
· **Side Plank** (pages 16–17)
· **T-Stabilization** (pages 20–21)
· **Fitness Ball Rollout** (pages 24–25)
· **Fitness Ball Hyperextension**
  (pages 26–27)
· **Hip Crossover** (pages 34–35)
· **One-Armed Sit-Up** (pages 38–39)
· **V-Up** (pages 42–43)

· **Reverse Crunch** (pages 44–45)
· **Penguin Crunch** (pages 50–51)
· **Leg Raises** (pages 56–57)

Warrior Workout
Challenges the diehard who wants to maximize core stability, strength, athleticism, and ab definition.
· **Plank-Up** (pages 14–15)
· **T-Stabilization** (pages 20–21)
· **Fitness Ball Atomic Push-Up**
  (pages 22–23)
· **Body-Weight Squat** (pages 30–31)
· **One-Armed Sit-Up** (pages 38–39)
· **V-Up** (pages 42–43)
· **Penguin Crunch** (pages 50–51)
· **Fitness Ball Seated Russian Twist**
  (pages 54–55)
· **Leg Raise** (pages 56–57)
· **Superman** (pages 58–59)

Athlete's Workout

This workout gears up your core for the rotational performance that many sports demand.

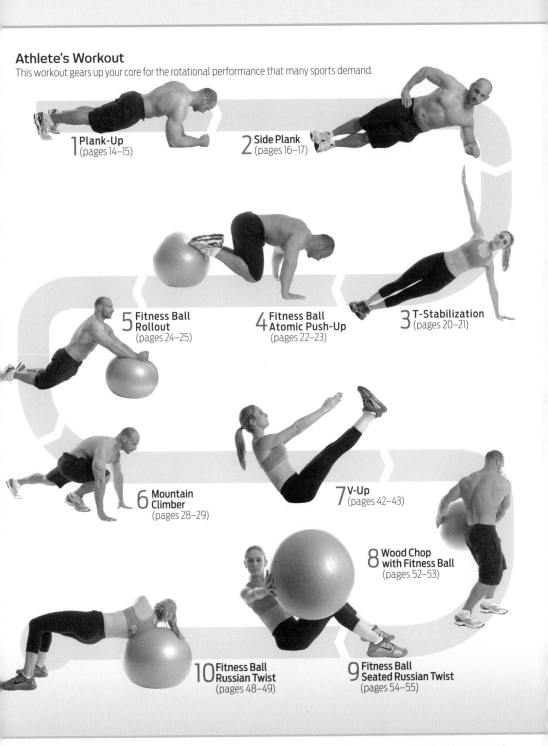

1 **Plank-Up**
(pages 14–15)

2 **Side Plank**
(pages 16–17)

5 **Fitness Ball Rollout**
(pages 24–25)

4 **Fitness Ball Atomic Push-Up**
(pages 22–23)

3 **T-Stabilization**
(pages 20–21)

6 **Mountain Climber**
(pages 28–29)

7 **V-Up**
(pages 42–43)

8 **Wood Chop with Fitness Ball**
(pages 52–53)

10 **Fitness Ball Russian Twist**
(pages 48–49)

9 **Fitness Ball Seated Russian Twist**
(pages 54–55)

About the Author

Hollis Lance Liebman has been a fitness magazine editor, national bodybuilding champion, and author. He is a published physique photographer and has served as a bodybuilding and fitness competition judge. As a Los Angeles resident, Hollis has worked with some of Hollywood's elite, earning rave reviews. Visit his Web site, www.holliswashere.com, for fitness tips and complete training programs.

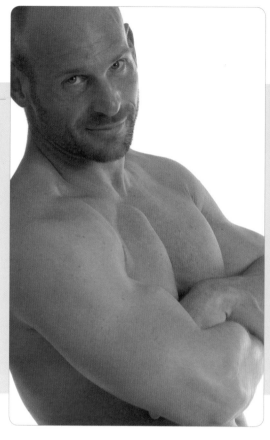

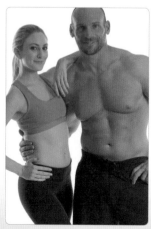

Core model Cori D. Cohen is a registered dietitian and healthy lifestyle coach based in New York City. She provides private nutrition counseling to a diverse clientele, in addition to working with residents at a nursing and rehabilitation center. Ms. Cohen has degrees from the University of Delaware, Fashion Institute of Technology, CUNY Queens College, and LIU C.W. Post. She has been currently featured as a columnist for the *Queens Courier*, where she provides readers with valuable nutrition advice.